Childhood Pain Stops Here

A Kids' Guide to SHOTS

Written by:

Robert M. Lowe, M.D., Ph.D.

and

Gina S. Lowe, J.D., Ph.D.

Copyright © 2018 Robert M. Lowe

All rights reserved.

ISBN: 978-1720865049

DEDICATION

This book is dedicated to a brave and courageous young boy named Griffin who learned to conquer his fear of shots and to be a role model for other kids with chronic conditions.

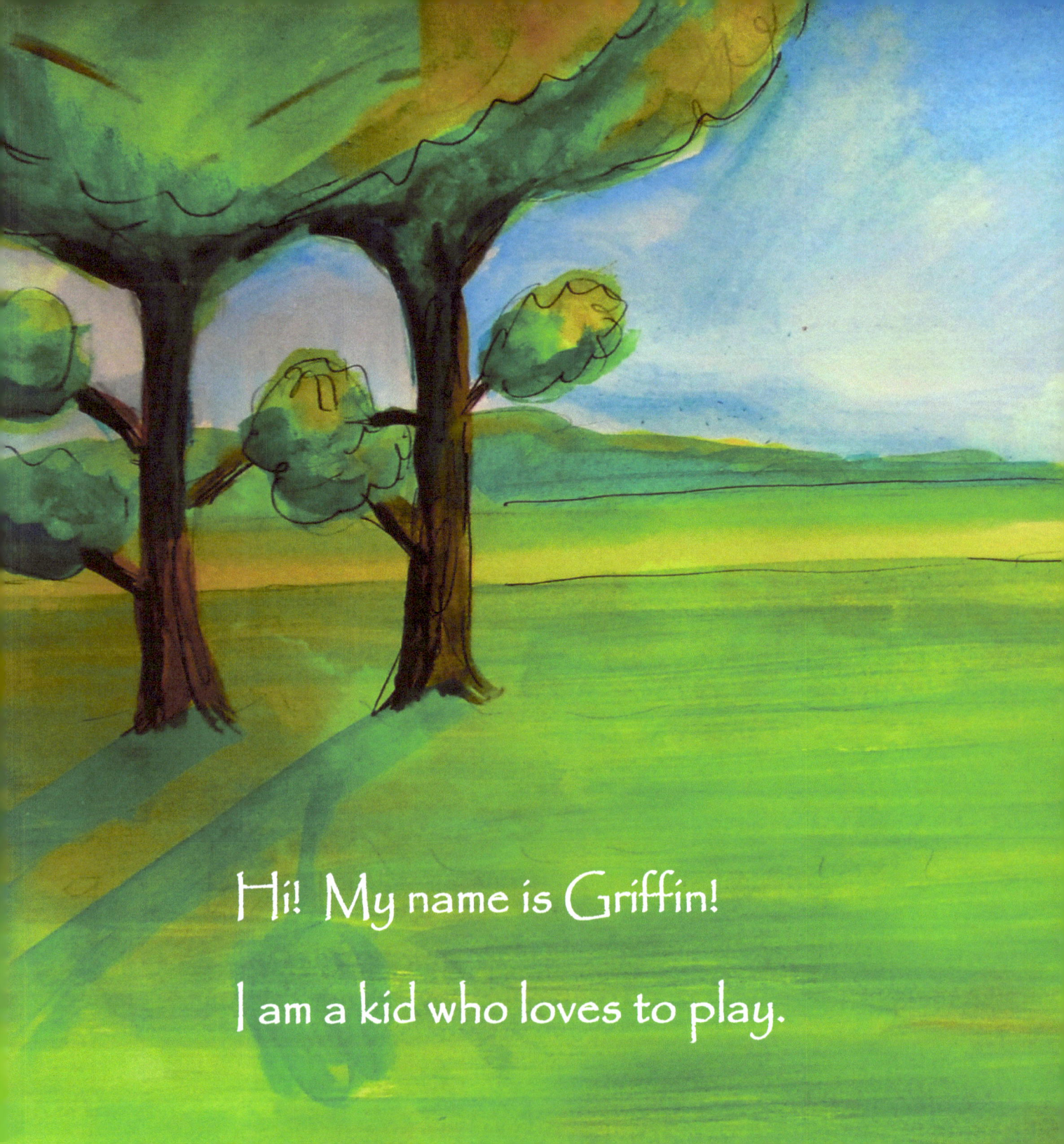

Hi! My name is Griffin!

I am a kid who loves to play.

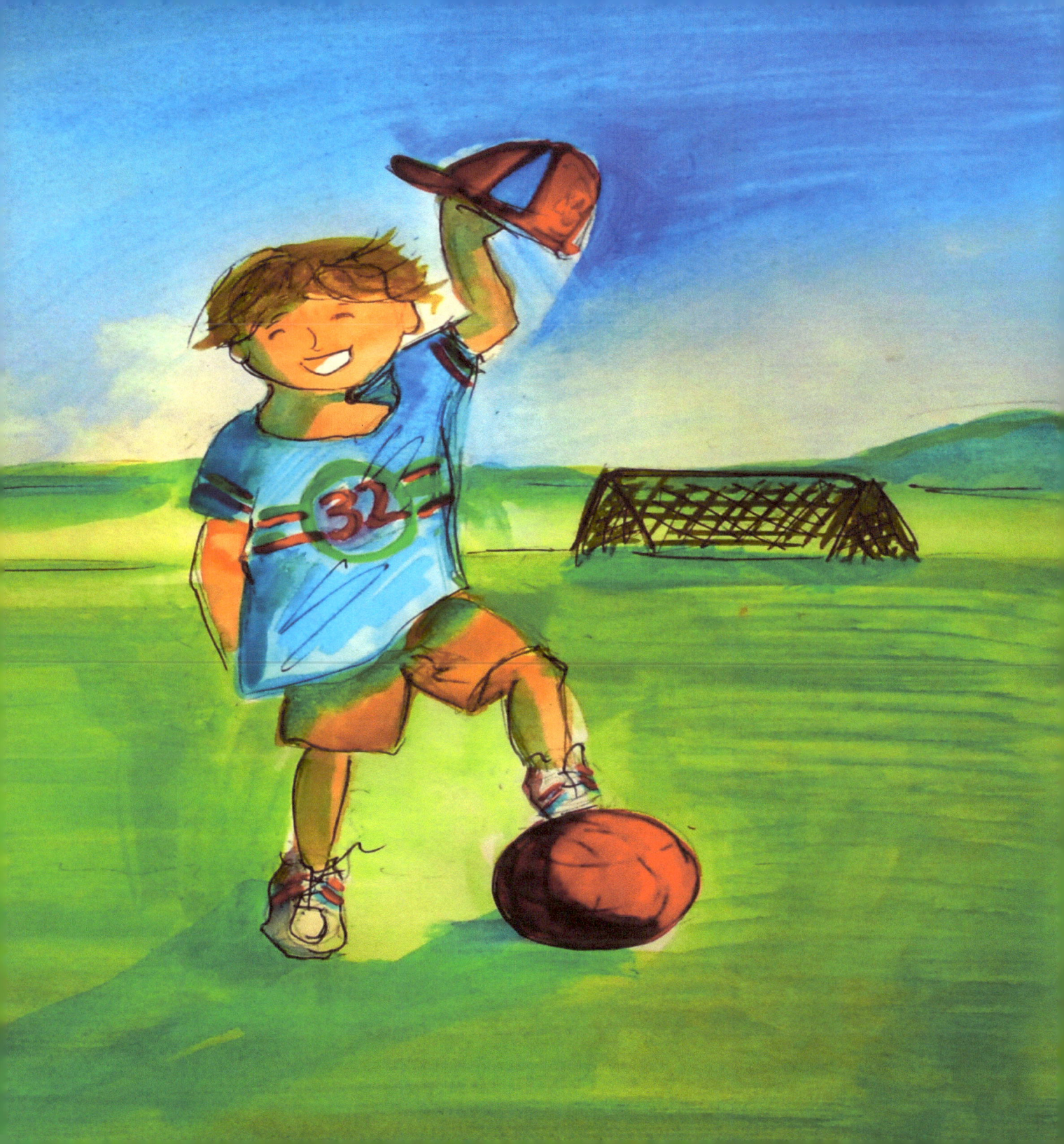

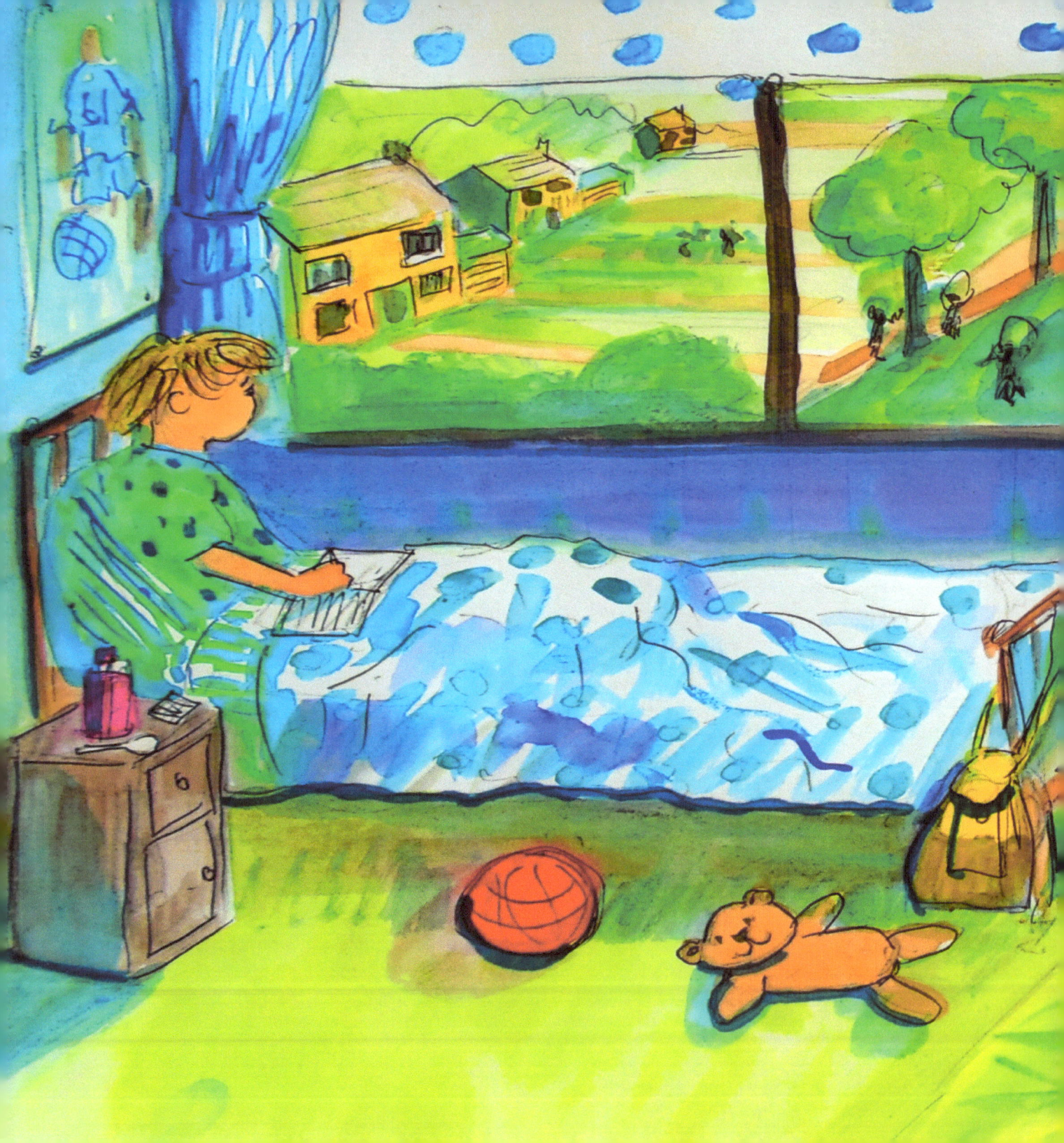

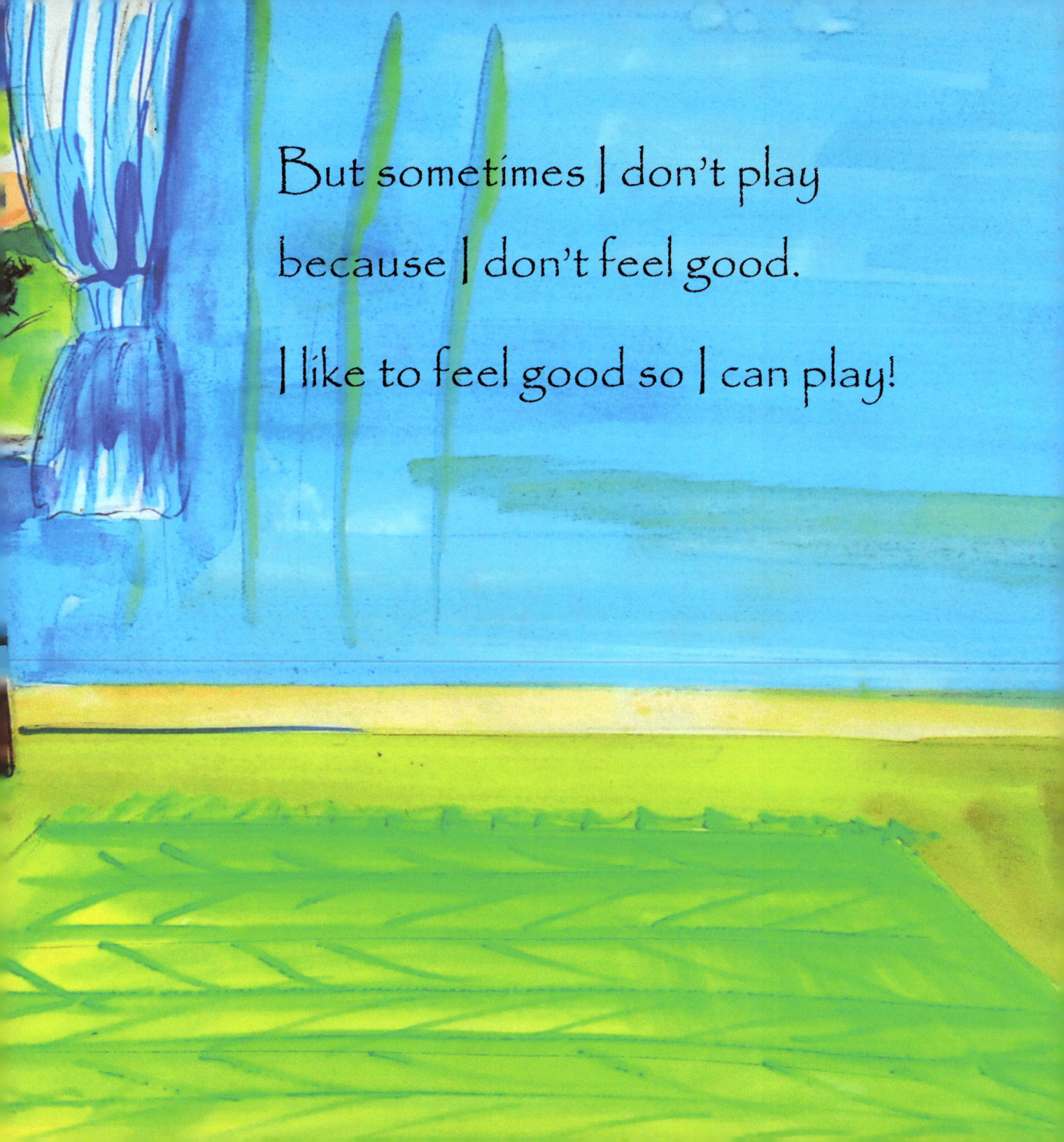

But sometimes I don't play because I don't feel good.

I like to feel good so I can play!

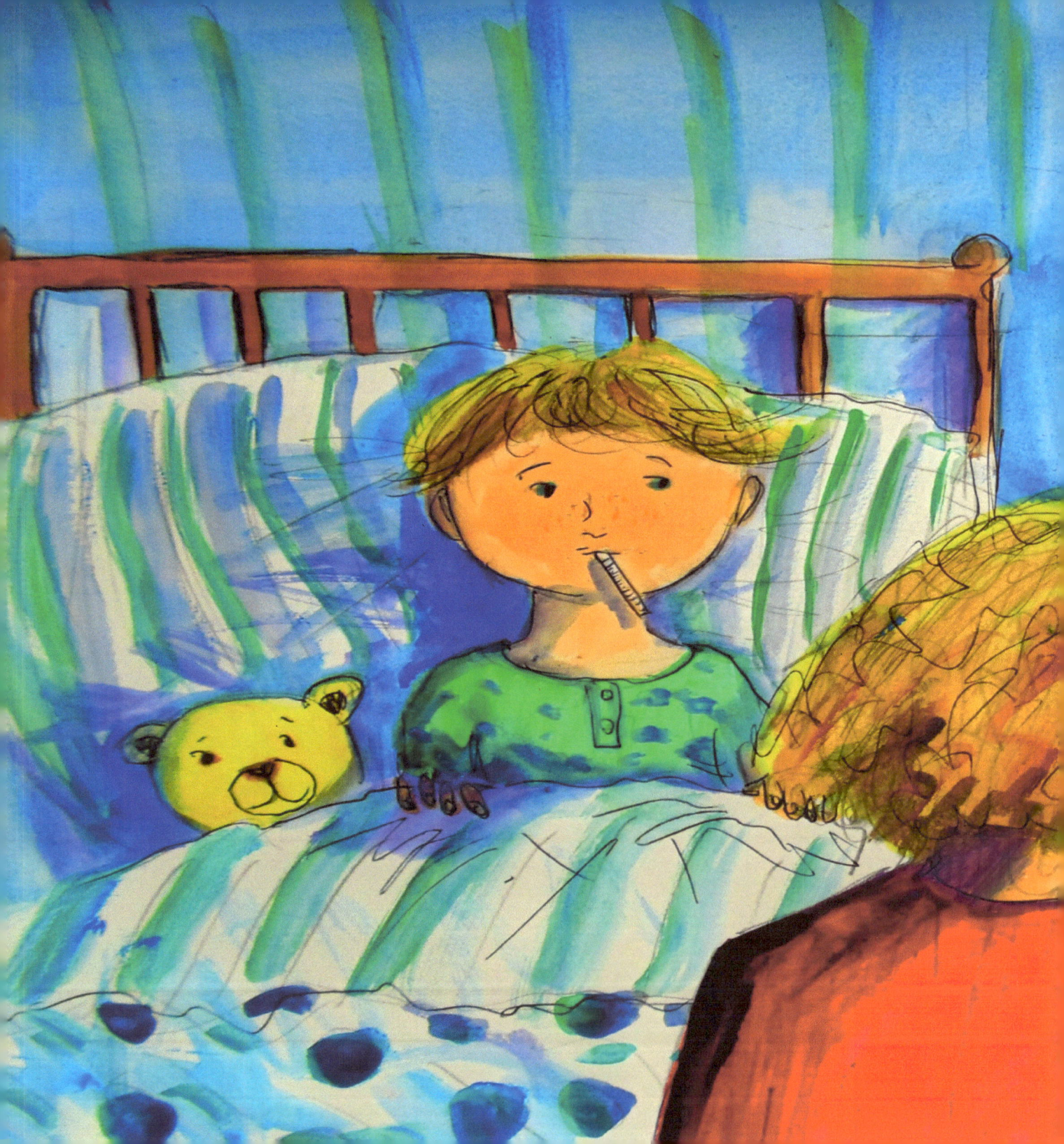

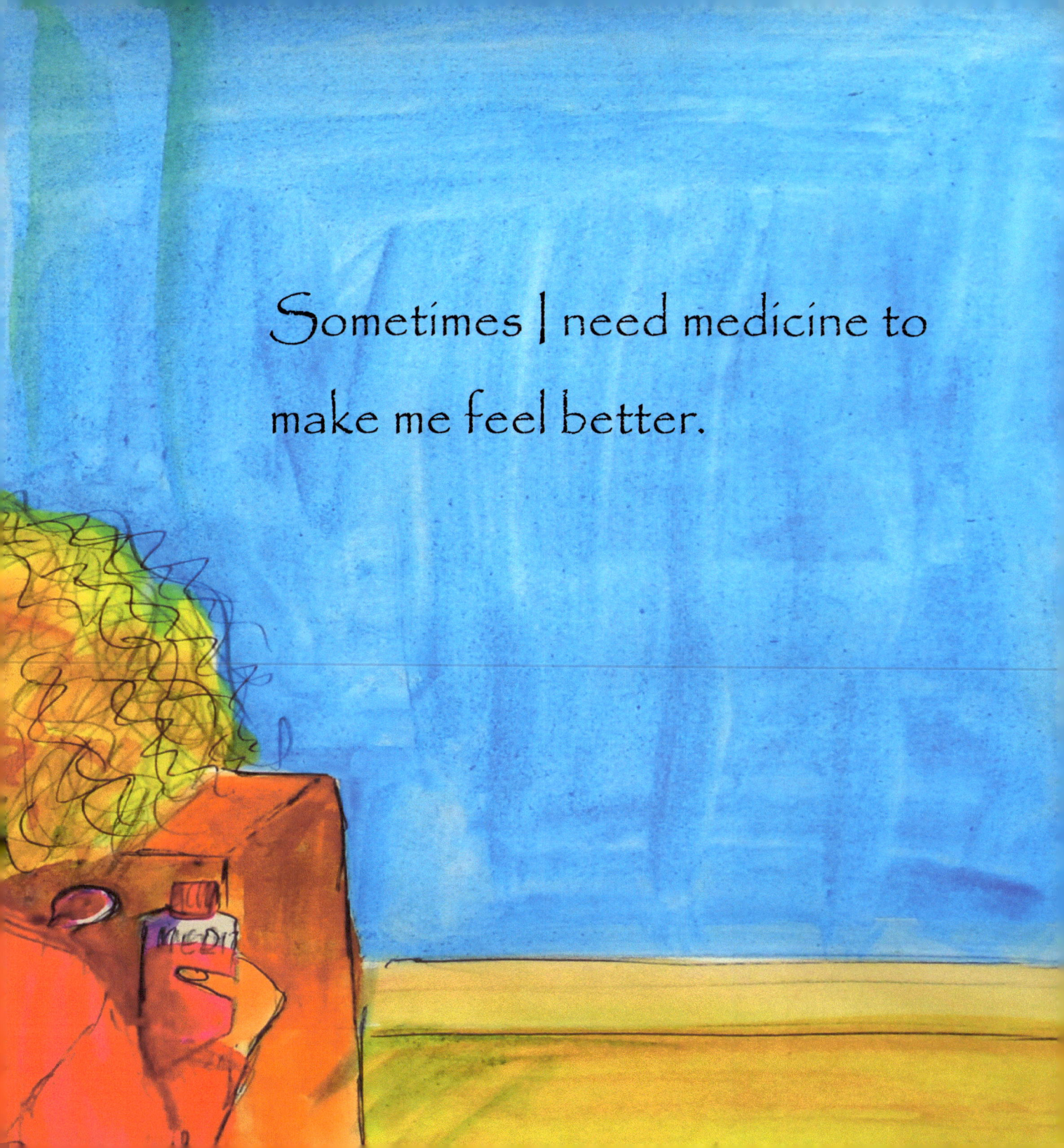
Sometimes I need medicine to make me feel better.

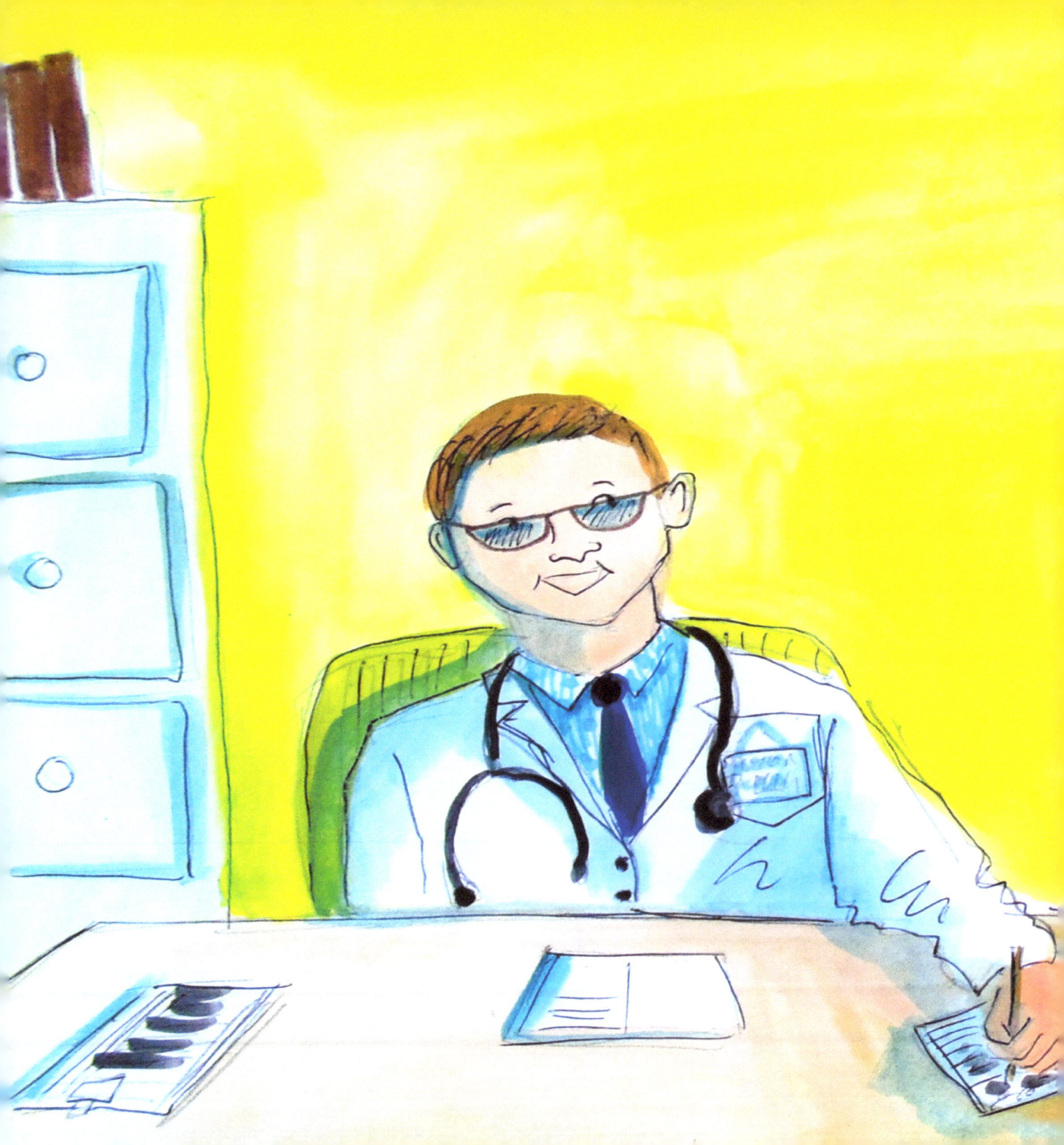

This is my doctor, Dr. Lowe, who cares about me and wants me to be happy. I am not happy when I don't feel good.

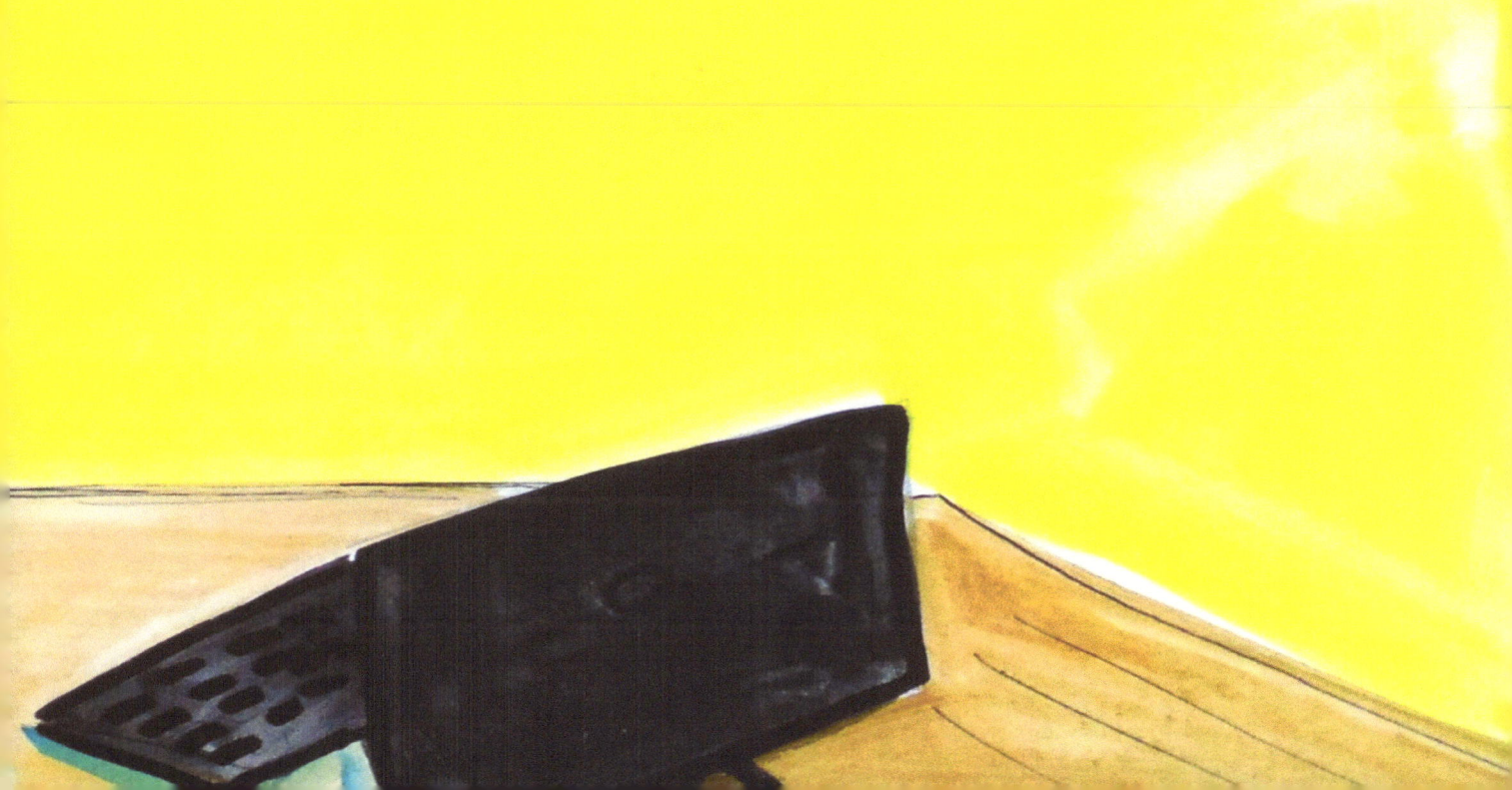

Sometimes Dr. Lowe tells me I need a shot. Shots are also called injections. The first time I needed a shot, I was scared. I know shots can hurt and it scared me.

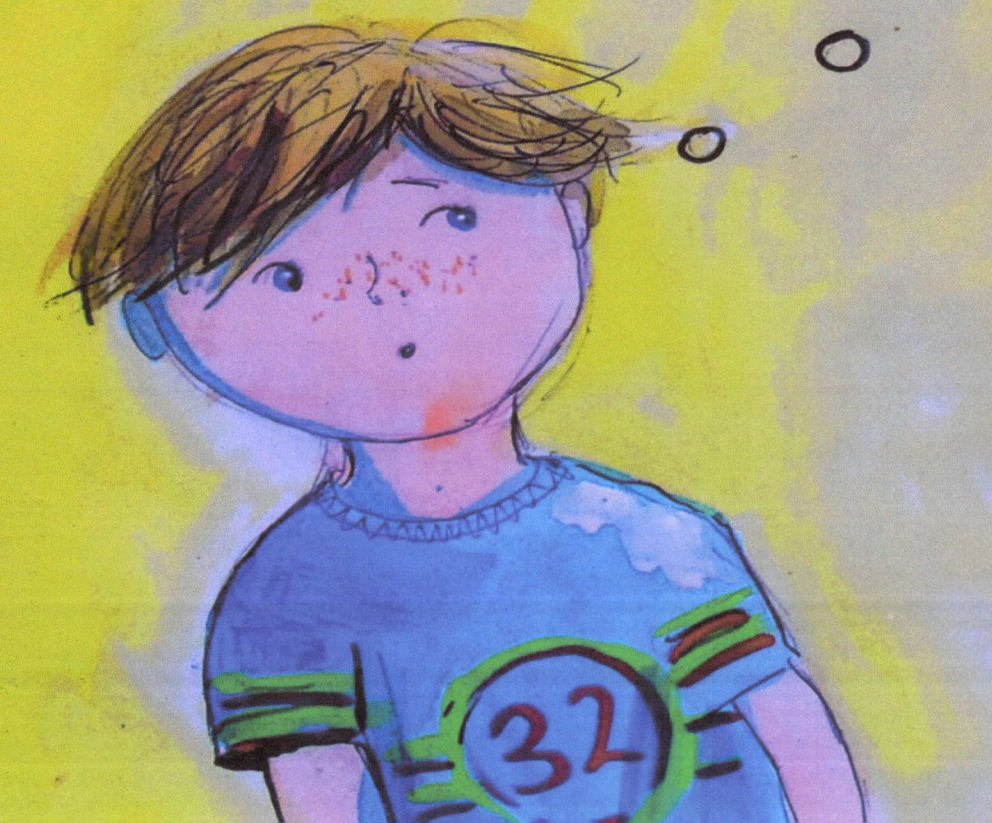

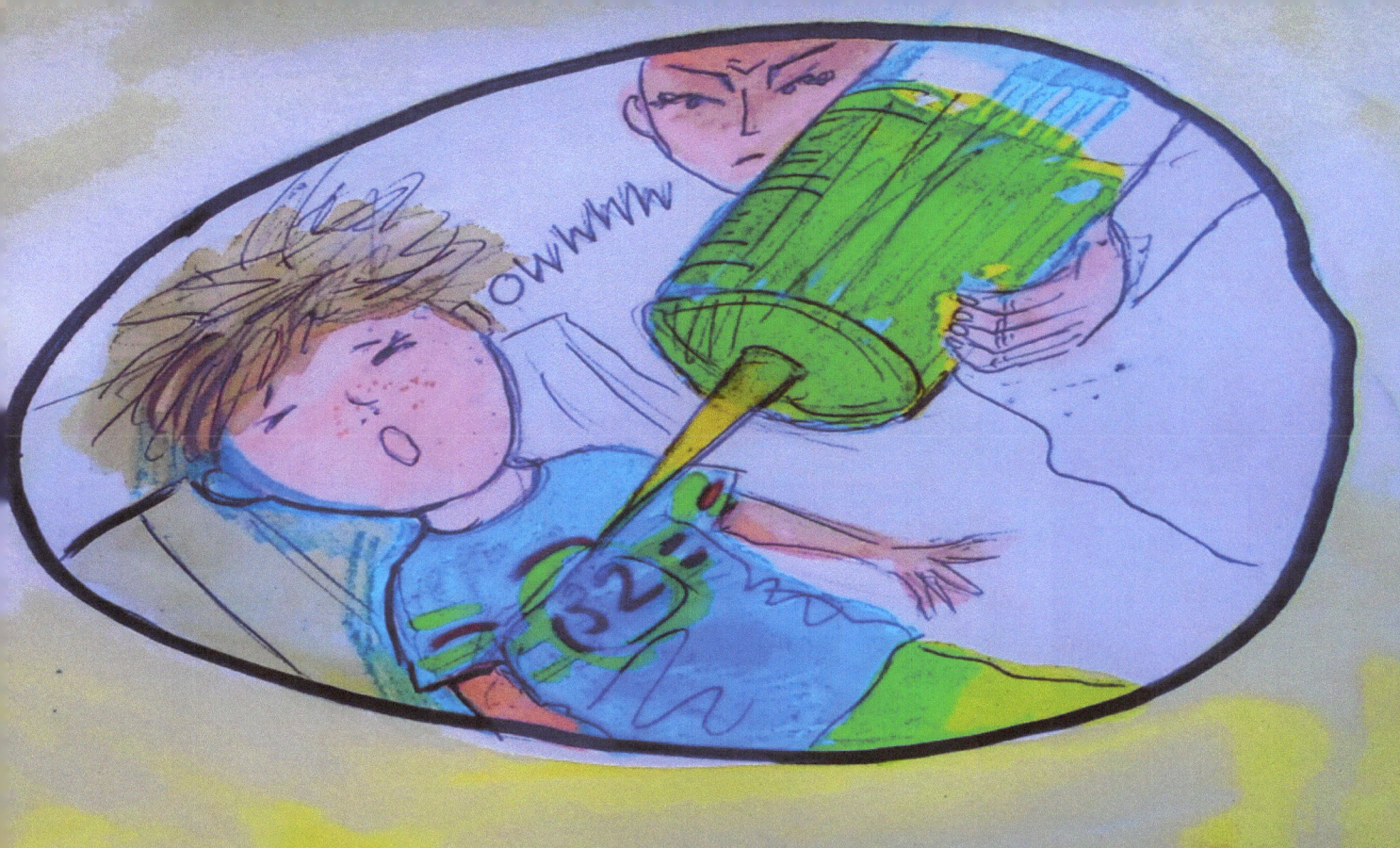

I did not want to get a shot. I was upset and worried, thinking about the shot. I imagined a giant needle. I imagined that I would have great pain from the shot.

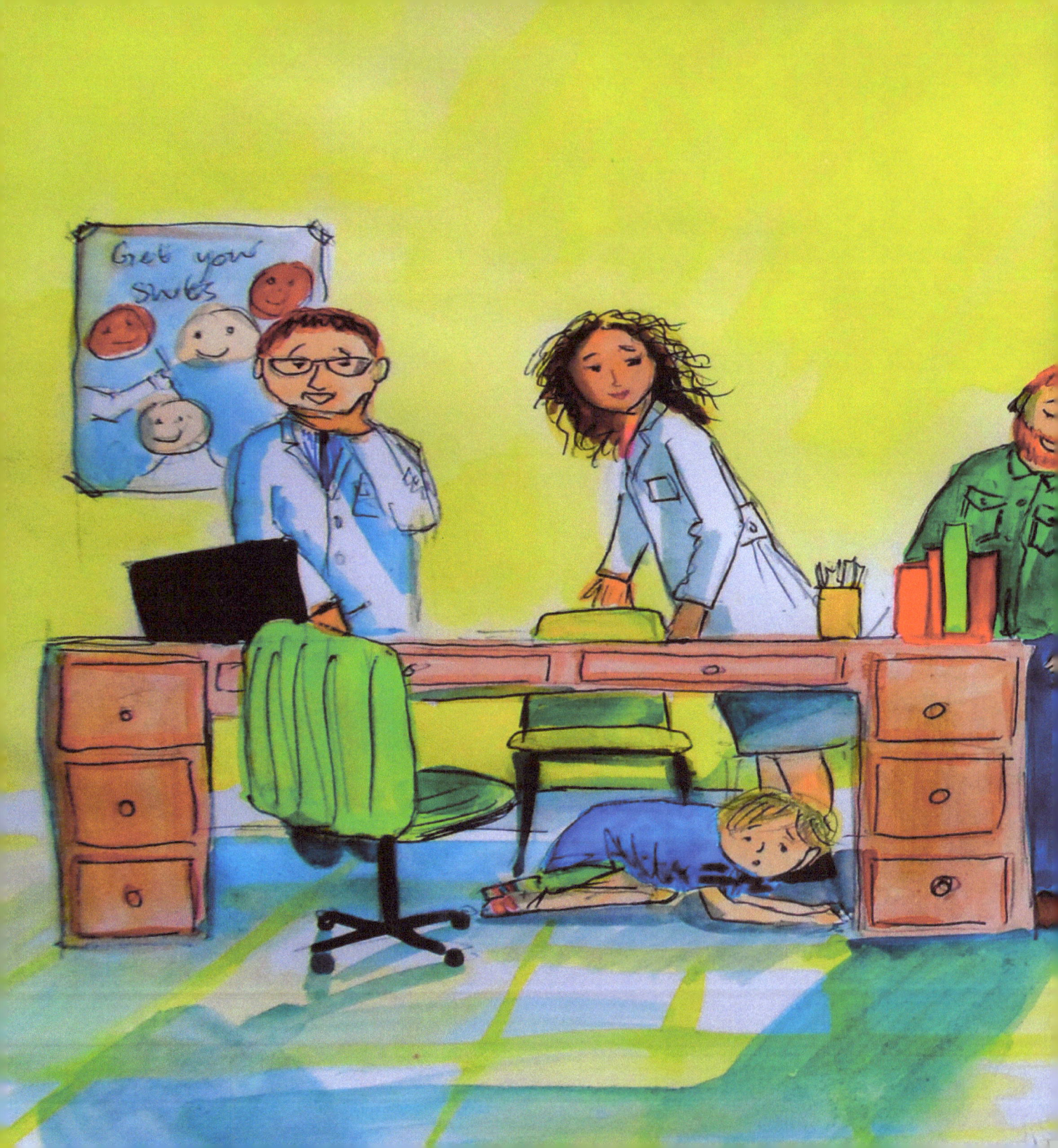

I was so scared, I wanted to run and hide under the table.

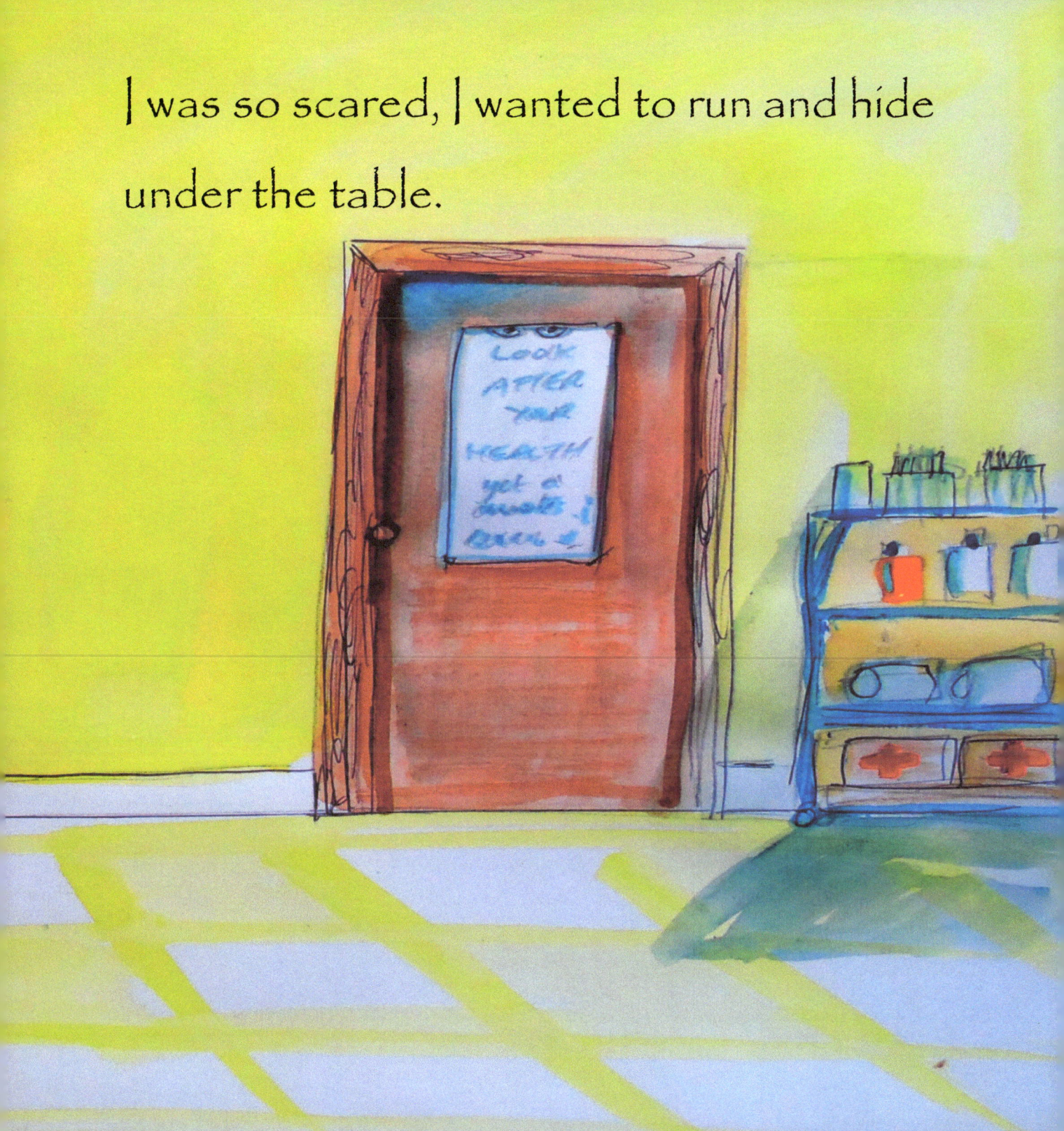

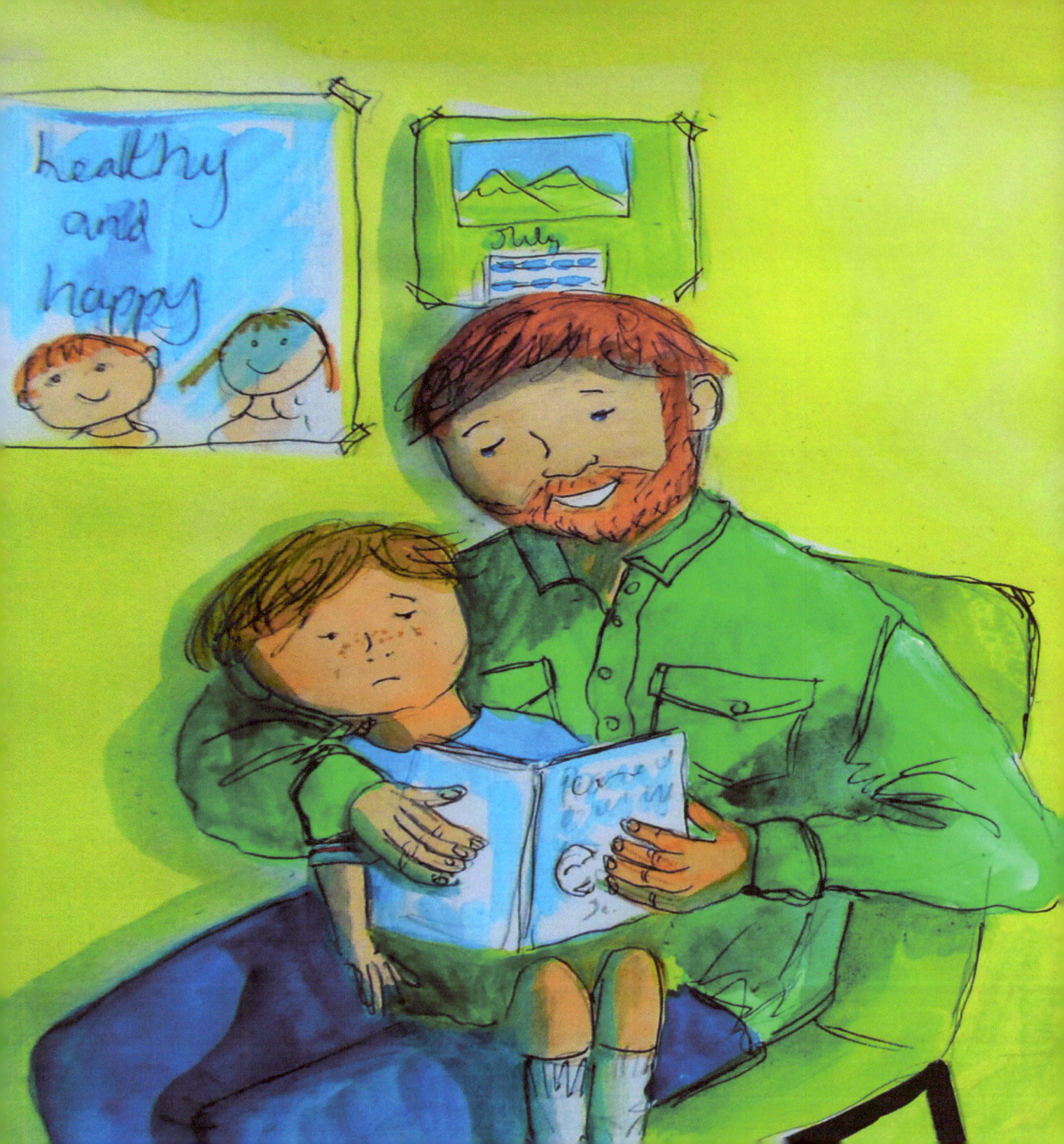

My dad hugged me and told me a story. He told me that there was a boy named Griffin who was in pain every day and could not play like the other kids. Griffin had pain that would not go away. Griffin was very unhappy that he hurt and could not play and have fun with the other kids. My dad explained that the shot would hurt a little, but not for long! Without the shot, the pain I was already feeling might not go away.

I wanted the pain to go away. I wanted to play. I wanted to feel my best. Although I was scared, I told my dad that I wanted to have the shot so I would feel better.

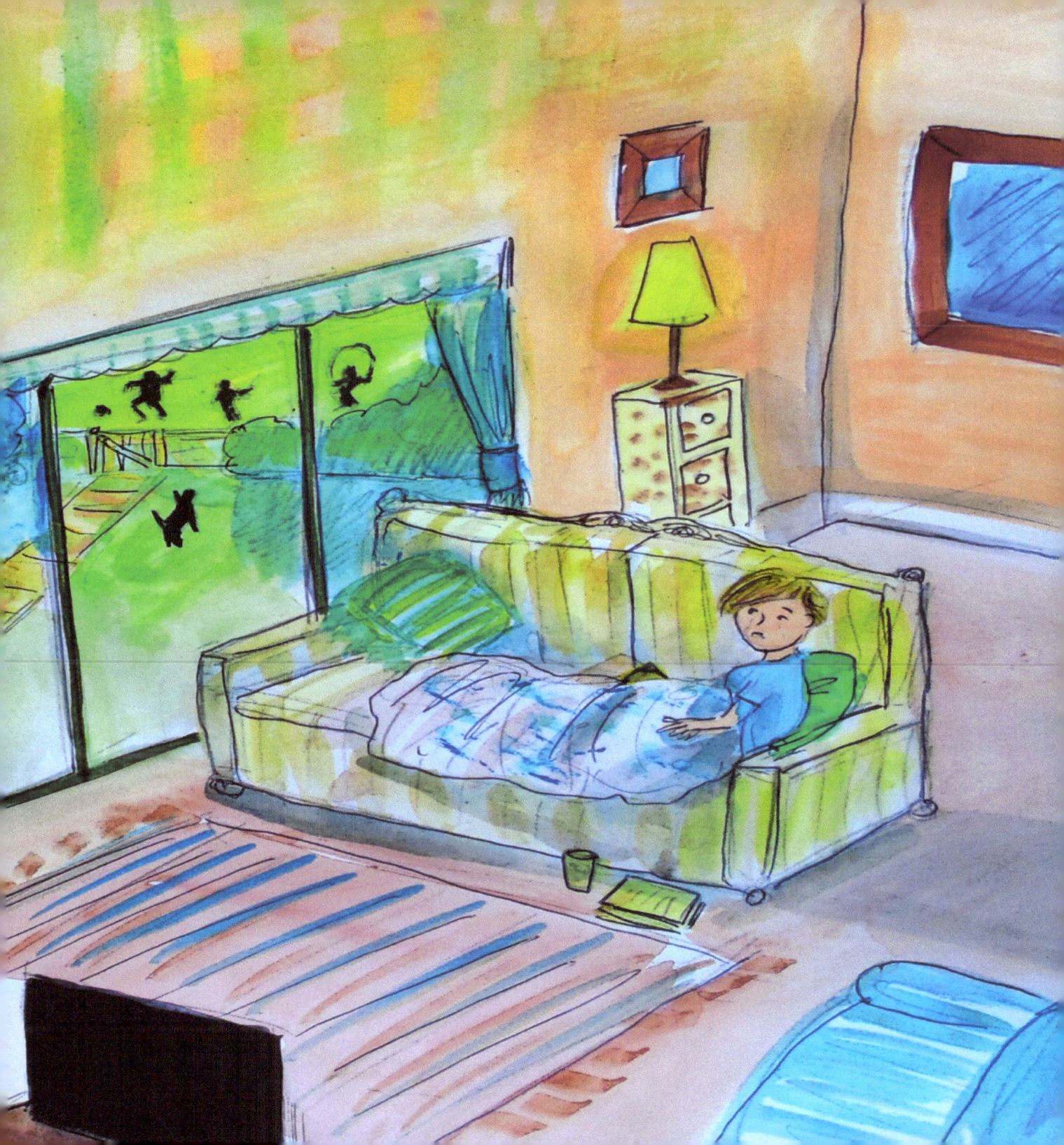

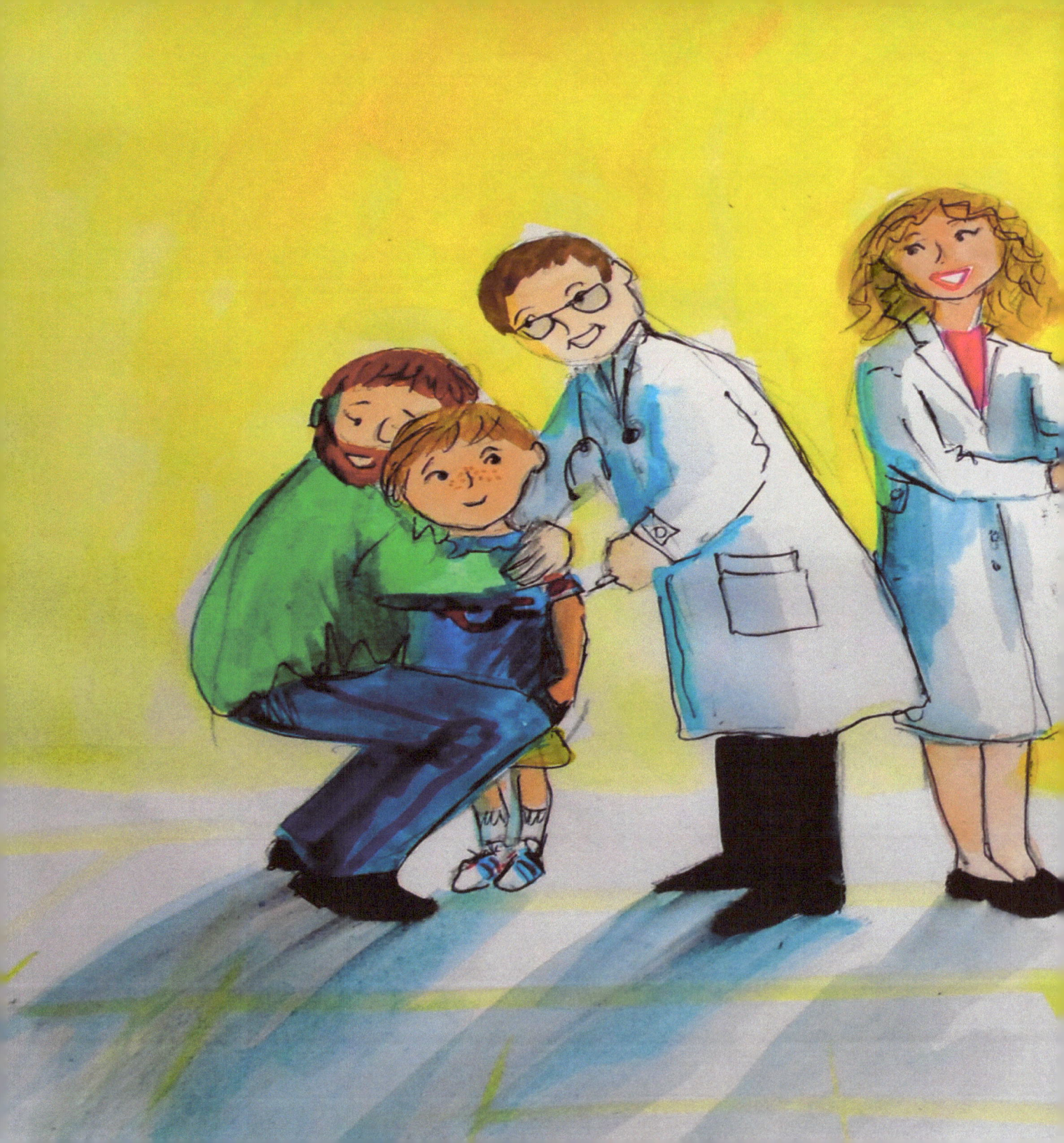

My dad smiled and hugged me tight. My dad was right and it did hurt a little. But the needle was a lot smaller than I expected. And the pain was over fast!

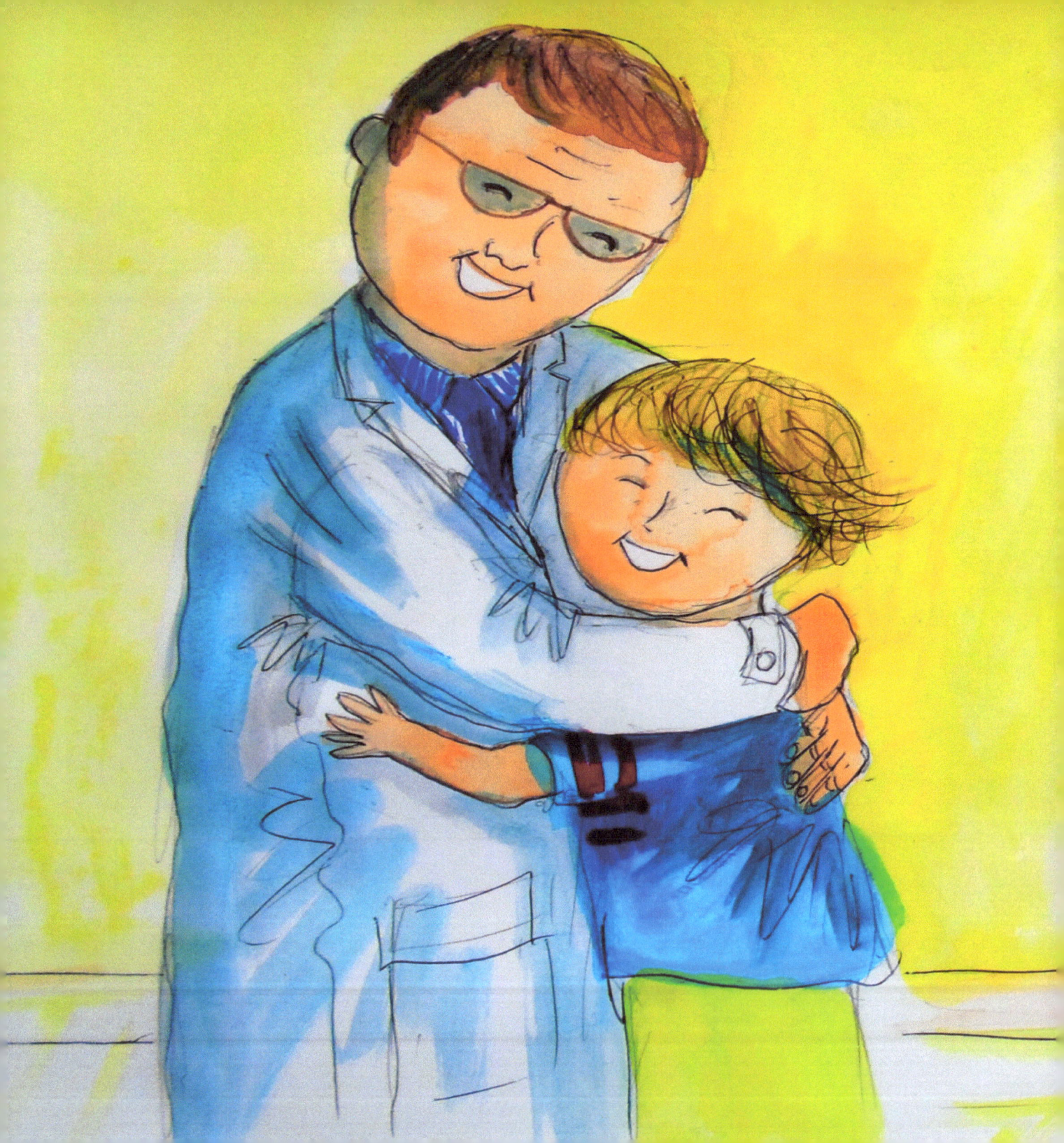

I got a big hug from Dr. Lowe and his assistant Rosie for being brave.

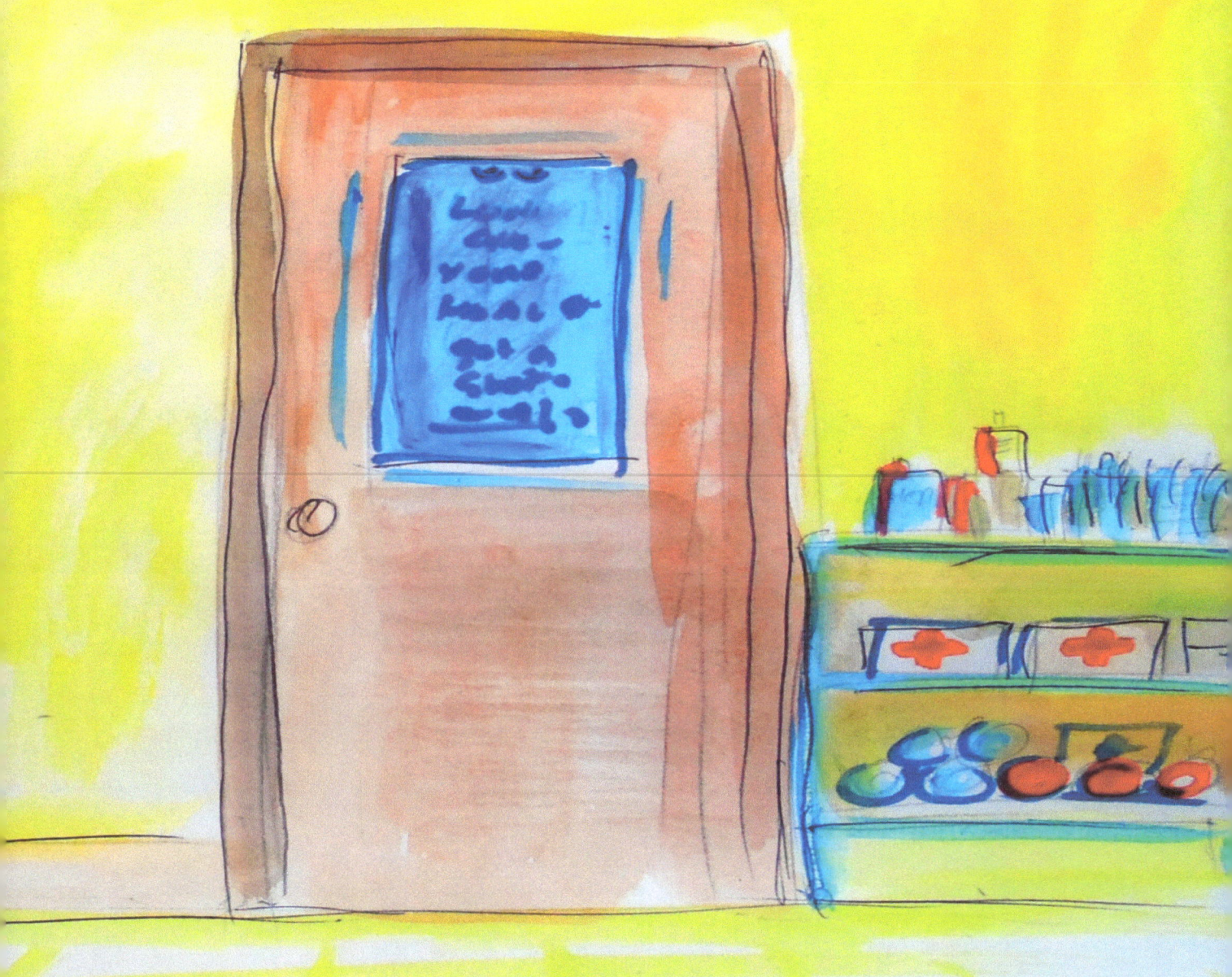

This is to certify that Griffin___ has been very Brave and this is a certificate of BRAVERY. Well done Griffin from Dr Lowe + Rosie

I am proud of myself! My dad is proud of me, too!

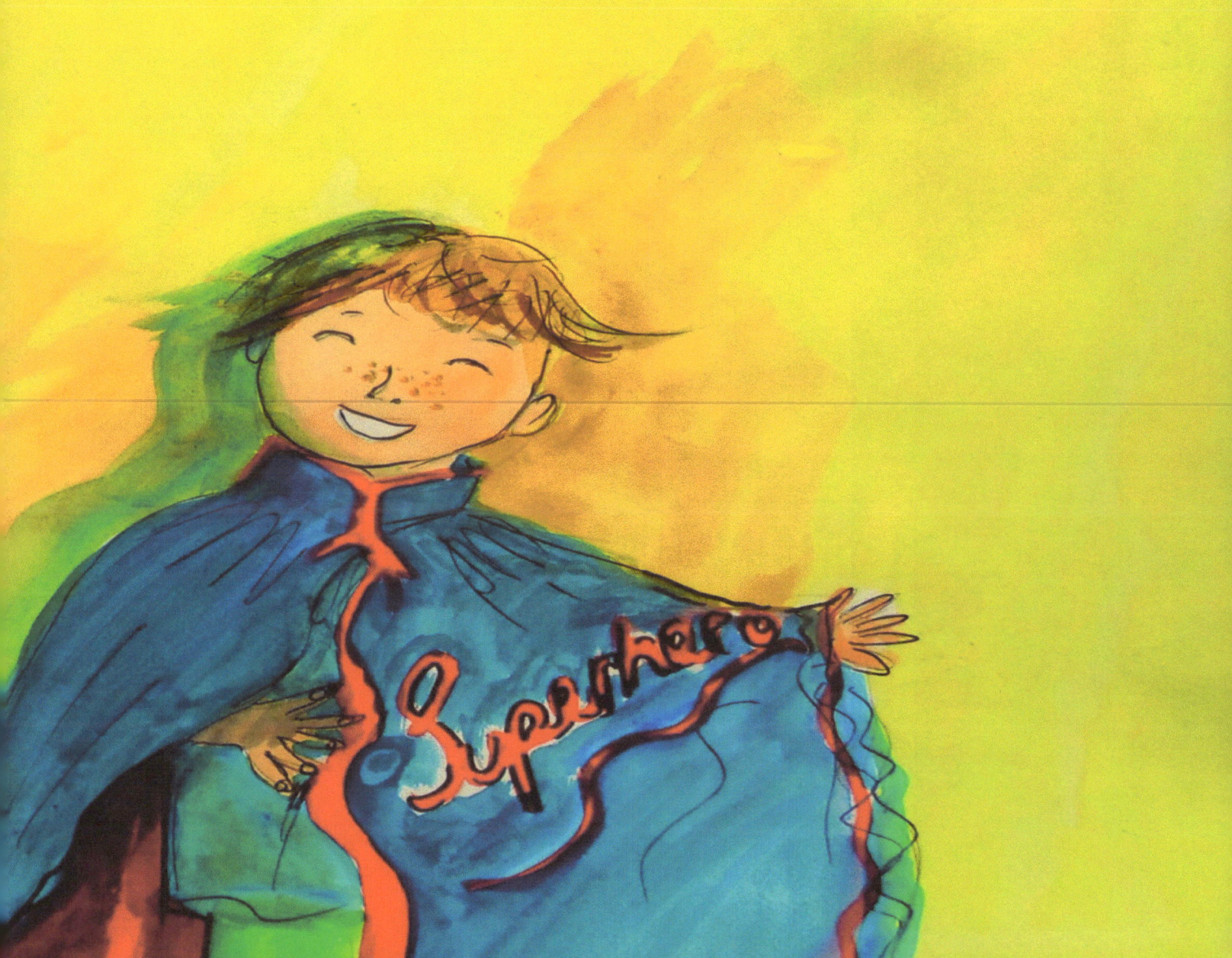

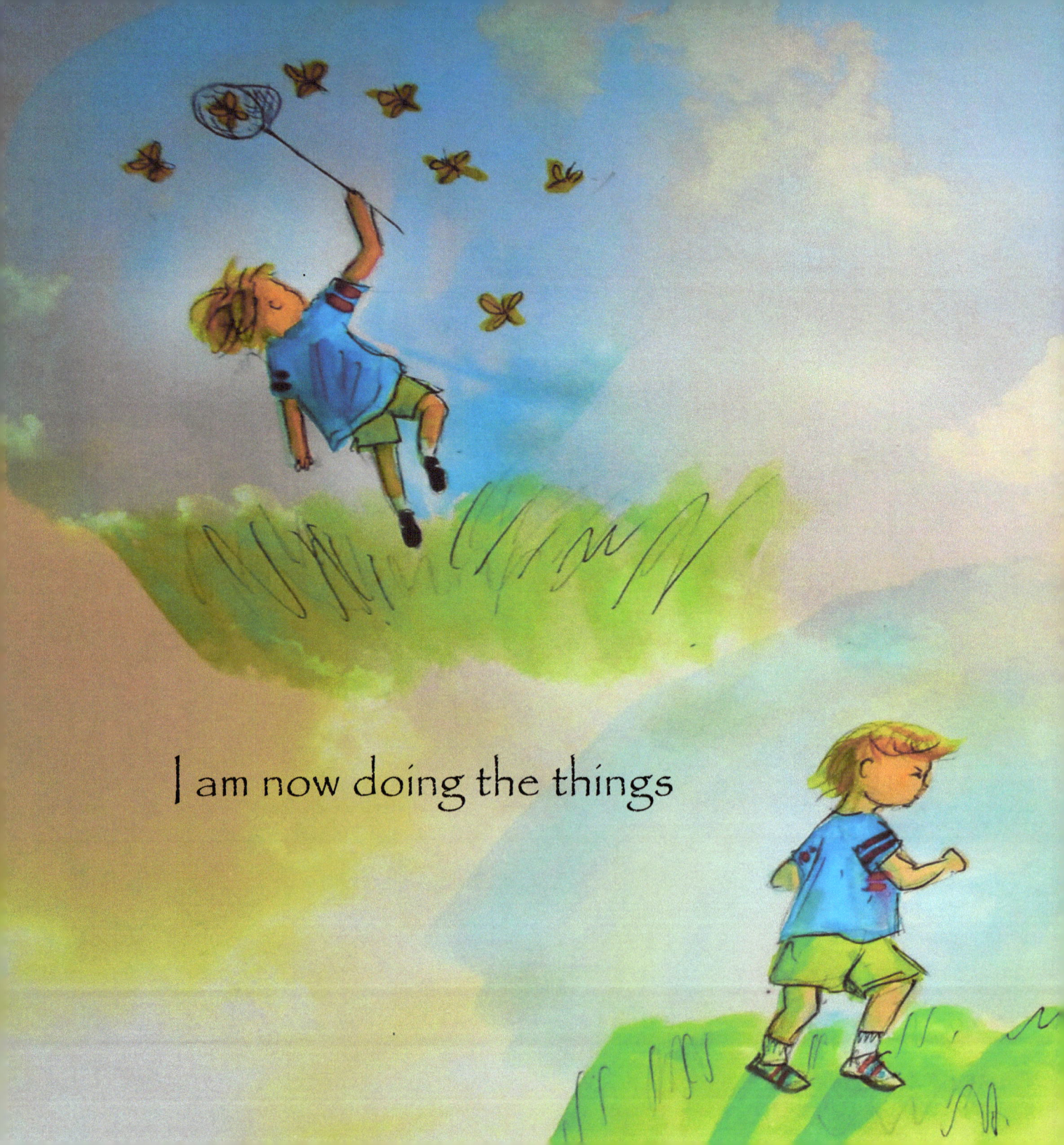
I am now doing the things

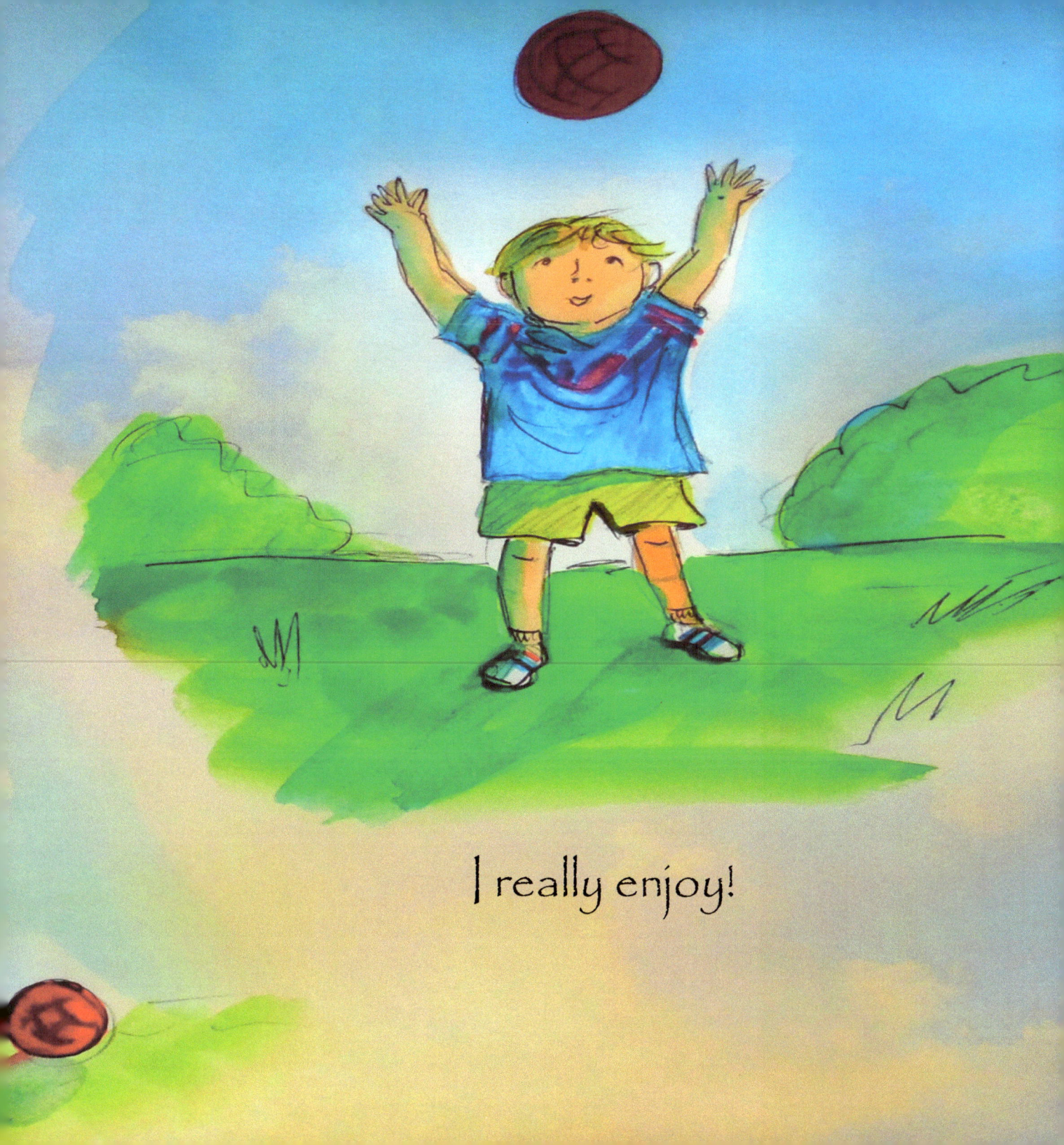

I really enjoy!

ABOUT THE AUTHORS

Dr. Robert Lowe is a pediatric rheumatologist who has dedicated his life to helping children, afflicted with chronic rheumatologic conditions, live pain-free lives. Dr. Gina Lowe is a child advocate who devotes her time to helping families to better understand chronic rheumatologic conditions.

www.ingramcontent.com/pod-product-compliance
Lightning Source LLC
Chambersburg PA
CBHW051829210526
45473CB00005B/1793